I0470391

We're Still Here

*Understanding, Caring and Supporting Seniors living
with Alzheimer's and Dementia*

Dr. Corie D. Johnson
CNA, CMT, MA, ALM

Copyright © 2019 (Dr. Corie D. Johnson)

All rights reserved

All rights to this book are reserved. No permission is given for any part of this book to be reproduced, transmitted in any form or means; electronic or mechanical, stored in a retrieval system, photocopied, recorded, scanned, or otherwise. Any of these actions require the proper written permission of the publisher.

This book is dedicated to all the women and men that have lost a loved one to this disease, I wish you well through this delicate journey of life. Continue to love, and comfort each other throughout this time of need. – C. Johnson

Contents

CHAPTER FIVE

DISCLAIMER

All knowledge contained in this book is given for informational and educational purposes only. The author is not in any way accountable for any results or outcomes that emanate from using this material. Constructive attempts have been made to provide information that is both accurate and effective, but the author is not bound for the accuracy or use/misuse of this information.

INTRODUCTION

Understanding the roles that seniors play in our societies and the beauty that they add to our environment is essential for us. They are an integral part of a nation, and I would want to believe that almost every family have a senior, either living with them or staying further away. Now let's pause there; have you ever thought about what it takes to be a senior? Do you ever wish to become a senior someday? With your present moment, have you ever thought or imagined what your senior phase of life would look like? If you can ponder on these questions, and take your time to read this book, then I believe you are on the right track towards understanding the seniors around you.

Becoming a senior could be somewhat challenging to seniors themselves, and also to people living around them; when they start noticing changes in their body that were not there before, but started springing forth along the line, the health issues they face while transitioning into the phase of a senior and how they are managing their senior status is worthy of note, having people around them at this moment of their lives to understand them, care for them, and support them is an act that would go a long way.

This book was written to bring awareness and educate people so that they could understand what it takes to be a senior, how to live peacefully and happily with a senior, and how to care and support for seniors while they are still with us without making them feel isolated in any way. I have also discussed extensively Alzheimer's disease and Dementia, which are two of the health conditions that affect seniors; how to understand the nature of these diseases, the effects, and control of Alzheimer's and Dementia, and how to care and support seniors living with these diseases. I would love you to flow with me as I take you through this journey of bringing clarification and understanding to the issues surrounding seniors.

The journey is eternal!

CHAPTER ONE
WHO IS A SENIOR?

Can you recognize a senior when you see one? When you hear people use the word Senior, who do you think they are talking about? Let me spare you too many questions and tell you who they are.

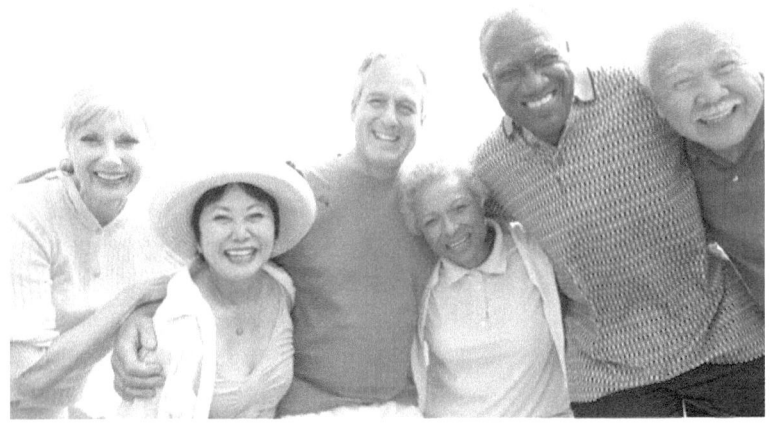

A senior, also known as senior citizens can be referred to as elderly persons. A senior citizen can be viewed from a social and demographic context based on the age bracket that they belong. You will agree with me that you cannot refer to a 40-year-old as a senior, that's someone actively working in full capacity. A senior is a person who has reached retirement age from work. Invariably, for you to be a senior citizen, you must have transitioned from being a working adult to becoming a retiree.

Traits of a Senior

There are certain traits that a person around you will exhibit that would make you know for sure that the person is a senior. Getting to identify a senior in our environment is not an arduous task in any form. From their appearance in physique, their carriage, the way they speak, and the way they handle happenings around them; you would deduce that these are seniors. The major outlined points below further describe the traits of a senior.

> ➤ *Experience and Accomplishments*

A senior is culturally seen as someone decelerating in their life, having accomplished a lot in life; from raising a family to having a career, and achieving major feats in their life. Seniors are experienced with life, wise and prosperous. What most seniors are known for is telling little children tales by the moonlight and stories of happenings when they were much younger. You can imagine having a senior that participated in the Second World War telling you about their experiences during the world war. If this person tells the story about life and that the war is no good, you have to listen to them, because they have seen it all; the good, the bad, and the ugly.

> ➤ *Medical Decline*

Medically, we can refer to a senior as one more prone to having to health issues, and most of the time these issues are age-related. This could be as a result of the fact that their body system is facing one form of degeneration or the other. The common health issues that they experience are usually in the form of hearing and vision impairment, dental problems, less efficient immune functions, sleep loss, urinary incontinence, and loss of mobility. Alzheimer's and Dementia are also major health issues affecting seniors that would be discussed with much emphasis in the later sections of this book. Seniors having one medical issue, or the other are more likely to suffer chronic pains most especially in the bones and joints, frequent illness, and frequently, they require people to give help and support to them. At this point in their life, proper care is all they need, because they don't have much time like they do before.

> ➤ *Economically Assisted*

Having known that a senior is a person retired from a paid active service and can no longer work, most seniors don't have a well-defined source of income to finance themselves. And as such, they require financial support which could be in the form of retirement funds, pension, savings, or financial support from caregivers. Their incapacitated nature brings them to become financially dependent on others for their well-being, and they are expected to be assisted to be able to cover their daily expenses and essential bills. Although, there are exceptions to those who had successful businesses and have more than enough in their reserves, with a lot of investment yielding a huge turnover for them.

➤ They Seek More Attention

One of the major traits you are going to discover about seniors is that they are always driven to seek more attention, at this point they take advantage of holding down anyone who comes around them for a visit. It is believed that they are always lonely at that phase of life. Whenever you visit a senior, they will always want to hold you down with their kind gestures, telling you stories and wanting to make you feel comfortable around them. Although, most times this doesn't work when it comes to dealing with the young adults, because they get bored easily at the company of a senior, only for the exception of a few ones. However, little children always enjoy the company of seniors because of it easier for them to understand each other. So, at this point, seniors take solace in the company of little children. I could remember a movie I saw a couple of years back titled Secrets of Jonathan Sperry; I observe from the movie noticed that Jonathan Sperry, a senior, was always enjoying the constant company the kids in his neighborhood and he was able to touch the lives of the kids positively through his company with them. You can see from here that the kids-senior relationship is a mutual one, a win-win I must say.

➤ Religiosity

From my experience in life, and with seniors, I can tell you for a fact that generally, seniors are always more religious than the younger ones, although, this varies with different cultures and traditions. 90% of seniors in the United States are somewhat religious. The Pew Research Centre's study conducted on black and white seniors established that 62% of those within the ages of 65 – 74 and 70% within the ages of 75 and above asserted that religion was vital to them when compared to 54% within the age range of 30 – 49. I guess you can see the unique variation from there. Pew Research also discovered that seniors in the age range of 65 and above, 87% of blacks and 75% of whites pray daily. In another study on the practice of religion among seniors, it was discovered that out of over 60 seniors examined, 25% read the Bible daily while over 40% watch religious TV stations. Well, we can say that their act of being religious is born out of the fact that they are getting closer to being with God. That's on a lighter note anyways.

The Senior Phase of Life

Getting to the senior phase of life comes a sense of realization of things happening in your body. You start to notice that there are some things that you do before effortlessly that now takes you extra effort to achieve. Can you imagine a footballer that was used to running around playing soccer, and some point discovered that he couldn't run like he used to anymore, couldn't take shots as he used to and his eyesight failing him on pitch and getting tired quickly; no one needs to tell him that he is becoming a senior and it is time to retire from the youthful activities. Also, a woman feeling all sexy with her boobs standing in the right angles, with ceaseless beauty, and a silky smooth skin would even realize that she is getting to the phase of a senior when she notices that those boobs that maybe was her selling point at those times making the men go crazy start to sag, and the silky smooth skin start to wrinkle.

Age is also another essential phenomenon that brings one to the realization that you are now a senior. If you could notice, I did not mention the age range of a senior from the beginning of this book, well so you know, that was intentional. I would love you know about the age phase of the life of a senior here. Now that you know, I would also like you to know that age of a senior varies widely in different contexts. In the context of government, you are considered a senior when you reach retirement age, and the standard retirement age in the United States is 66, while in Canada it is 65, although they are gradually increasing to 67 in both countries. However, at age 62, you are eligible for social security benefits, but you can enjoy a senior discount if you visit McDonald's or Arby's and you around 55 years old. Also, once you turn 55, your data begins to enter the senior age demographic group. Looking at these different age range, we can tell that there is no crucial factor to determine what you must be to become a senior; although the age range listed above could tell more than you either become a senior or you have become a senior. So, if you are running around feeling like a minor, check your age in line with the age range listed above and you will realize that is not so anymore, you are now a senior. Understanding your senior phase of life in line with your age is crucial for you to know the best way to manage your body when you or your loved ones get to these age range.

The Health challenges that the body is faced with also tells more about the body transition into the senior phase of life. If you start to notice that you are frequently visiting the hospital for health issues like osteoarthritis and osteoporosis, dental problems, presbyopia, organ dysfunction, urinary incontinence, weakened vocal cords, Alzheimer's, Dementia, and other re-lated health issues; you should get conscious for sure that you or your loved ones are becoming a senior or are already a senior, and at this point proper attention and care should be given to your body, or better still you must take proper care of your seniors when you notice these changes in their health.

The funny thing you should understand is when a senior gets to that phase of consciousness that they are not an active adult anymore, but a senior, they are always faced the challenges of having to accept their new stage of life and make peace with it. It might be difficult for some people, most notably those whose lifestyle is surrounded with what they do as an active adult; examples are sportsmen and other celebrities that have al-ways enjoyed the spotlight, the aging transition might take them off the spotlight that they have always enjoyed all their lives. Looking at it from another angle, some people find it easy to make peace with the realization of their transition into the new phase of life without any issues.

CHAPTER TWO
ALZHEIMER'S AND THE SENIORS

In the old age of the seniors living around us, one of the challenges they are faced with is a decline in their health. During this phase of their lives, different diseases spring up, and worthy of note among them is Alzheimer's disease. Have you heard of Alzheimer's before? How well can you describe Alzheimer's disease? And how can you relate it to the seniors living around you? All these questions will be answered one after the other in this section. Let move on with this, shall we?

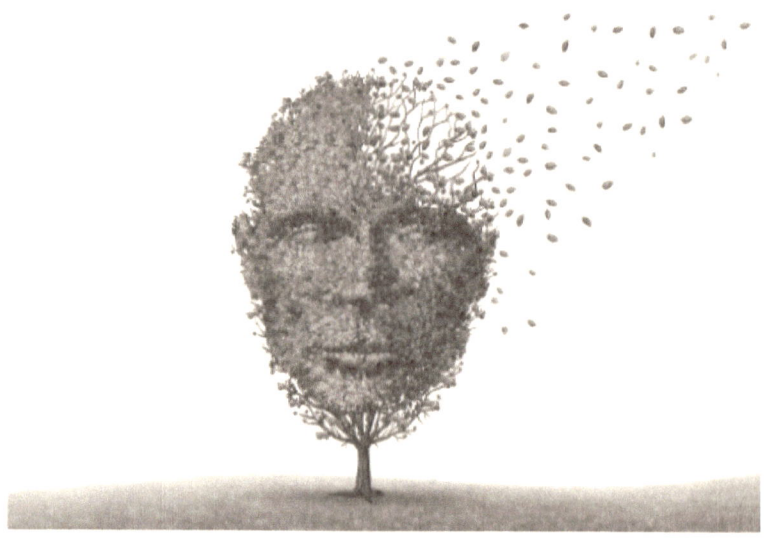

Understanding Alzheimer's Disease

So, let me tell you a bit about this disease so that you could get a more unobstructed view of it and a complete understanding. The thing is, the brain has 100 billion nerve cells called neurons. Each of these nerve cells connects with many other nerve cells to form communication networks. These nerve cells are formed into groups, and each group has their peculiar duties, which involves learning, thinking, smelling, remembering, feeling, hearing, among others. They receive supplies, they generate energy, get rid of waste, process and store information, and communicate with other cells. In short, they work like factories. Now, what Alzheimer's dis-ease does to the well-coordinated brain cells is it prevents part of the cell's factory from working well, thereby causing gradual damages and break-downs in the brain cells. As the damage spreads, the cells lose their ability to work in full capacity and eventually dies causing irreparable damages to the brain. The symptoms now become evident in the outward coordination of the human with the disease.

Alzheimer's is one disease that is common among seniors. It is a form of a neurological disorder that causes degeneration and the death of brain cells, thereby resulting in memory loss and other cognitive abilities severe enough to affect daily activities of human life. Alzheimer's starts slowly with the condition gradually becoming worse over time which will lead to death sooner or later. It causes 60-80% of the cases of Dementia, which will be discussed in the later part of this book.

We cannot say for sure that Alzheimer's is a normal part of aging, but the notable among the risk factors of Alzheimer's is increasing age as many people affected are within the age range of 65 years and older. In the United States, approximately 200,000 of the people under the age range of 65 have the younger-onset version of Alzheimer's, which is also known as early-onset Alzheimer's. This figure just showed a minute one out of the massive number of Alzheimer's dominated among those who are 65 years and above.

Research has shown that in 2013, 6.8 million people in the United States were diagnosed of Dementia, and these people had a diagnosis of Alzheimer's; and by 2020, these numbers are expected to be doubled. That's something serious there I must say. I guess we are going to leave the research on better ways to reduce and minimize the effects to our sci-entists, who I believe have been working tirelessly on that. What we are concerned with here is to understand how the disease operates among the senior, and ways of managing this disease.

Associated Symptoms

You will see obvious signs, and when you see these symptoms occurring in you or your loved ones that are seniors, be sure that there is a presence of Alzheimer's in that body. But it is of importance for you to know that the most common symptom of Alzheimer's is difficulty in remembering newly learned information; when you just informed your loved one about something, and some moments later you asked them about the earlier information you shared with them, it is possible that they forget or even argue with you that you never said that. When you notice this, don't take offense, understand that it is as a result of Alzheimer's.

It could be likened to the rest of our bodies, and our brain encounters some changes as we age. Most of us sooner or later notice some slowed thinking and occasional issues with bringing certain things to remembrance; severe memory loss, getting confused at pieces of stuff, and other significant changes in the way our minds work may be a sign that the brain cells are failing.

Alzheimer's changes start in the part of the brain affects learning. As this disease develops through the brain it goes deeper to causing more severe symptoms, which includes disorientation, mood, and behavior changes; more profound confusion about events, time, and place; unfounded suspicions about family, friends, and professional caregivers; and difficulty in speaking, swallowing and walking.

We have over time noticed that people having symptoms of Alzheimer's usually find it difficult to accept the fact that they have a problem. Although, along the line as the situation worsens, they realize the need to get diagnosed and get the necessary care to manage the disease.

The symptoms of Alzheimer's are generally categorized into three stages:

1. Early Stage Alzheimer's

In the early stage of Alzheimer's, the signs that will be noticed include the following:

- ***Difficulty in remembering episodes of forgetfulness:*** Here you will state forgetting things by default when you learn new stuff, it doesn't stick to your brain; hence you will not remember.

- *Forgetting names of family members or friends:* You will see your old-time buddy that has always rocked with you for years, and you will find it difficult to remember their names. I could recall a senior I stayed with a few years back having the issue of placing the name of his niece with her identity. This is funny but serious.

- *Some confusion in situations outside the familiar:* This involves you finding it difficult to recognize the areas that you usually go through, you could even get missing in your neighborhood, in which you have lived for years. That's how bad it could be.

2. Middle Stage Alzheimer's

The middle stage of Alzheimer's is identified with the following symptoms:

- *Deepened confusion in many circumstances:* Now at this stage, the level of complexity is getting worsened, and you tend to lose your sense of judgment on specific issues.

- *Trouble recognizing locations:* Alzheimer's patient finds it difficult to identify places they have been before and passed through severally; this is more intense in this stage than the earlier stage.

- *Problems with sleep:* At this point, the sleeping patterns becomes inconsistent, and sometimes, you find it difficult to sleep.

- *Greater difficulty with remembering recently learned information:* Knowledge that has been gathered recently tend to get faded in the memory lane. You start forgetting things that you had learned years before the disease became evident.

3. Late Stage Alzheimer's

The late stage of Alzheimer's disease is comprised of the following symptoms:

- *Problems with speech:* At this stage, people with Alzheimer's starts to have a speaking impairment; they don't get to talk properly.

- *Poor thinking ability:* This disease affects the thinking faculty, with the inability to put thoughts straight and right.

- ***Unnecessary repetition of conversations:*** You keep saying things repeatedly till it becomes incoherent and doesn't make sense.

- ***Paranoia:*** This comes with a sense of feeling insecure around people, even your family members, and loved ones. It could lead to anxiety and being more abusive.

Diagnosis of Alzheimer's Disease

When all these symptoms that are known for Alzheimer's are noticed in you or in your loved ones that seniors, of whom are the principal focus in this book, it is crucial for you to book an appointment with the doctor for a proper diagnosis to be done, and taking care of the situation follows immediately.

The diagnosis of Alzheimer's does not require a particular test that is a must-do to know if one has it or not; what the doctors do is they check for the vital signs and symptoms of the disease, take a look at your medical history, and rule out every other conditions; after ruling out other possible conditions, the doctor will carry memory and cognitive tests, to look into the patient's ability to think and remember, before they make a diagnosis.

The doctors also look out for the patient's neurological function, for example, by testing their balance senses, and reflexes. Other assessments that may be carried out include a blood or urine test, CT scan, MRI scan of the brain, and screening for depression.

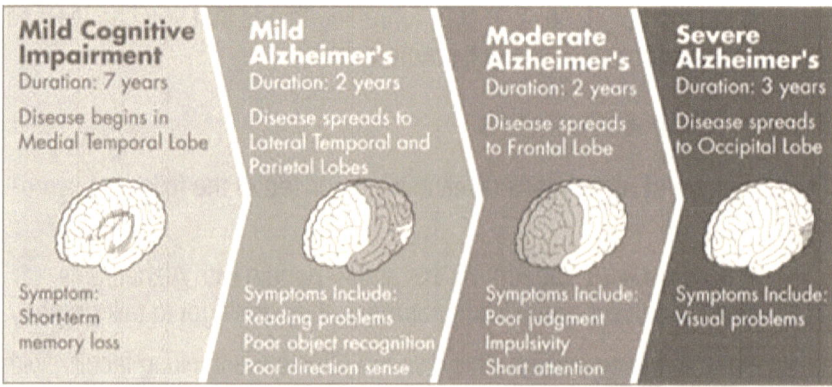

To ascertain that a person has Alzheimer's, there must be a visible presence of a gradual memory loss or a progressive cognitive impairment. So, the doctors do a cognitive assessment on the patients by asking the following questions:

- What is your age?
- What is the year?
- What is the time, to the nearest hour?
- What is the name of the hospital where you are present?
- What is your date of birth?
- Can you recognize these people, for example, a family, the doctor, the nurse, or a caregiver?
- Who is the president of your country?
- What is your address?
- Repeat an address of the test that I will give you now (for example, 21, Kensington drive).
- Count in descending order from 20 down to 1.

The way and manner these questions are answered will make the doctor give a correct diagnosis on the state of the disease; whether the condition is present at all, or the stage of the disease, if present.

Effects of Alzheimer's Disease on the Seniors

The disease of Alzheimer's affect a lot about the seniors living around us in the sense that it causes a total change in the seniors affected by the disease, if you have not seen a senior close to you in a while, and by chance you get to see them but they are already a victim of Alzheimer's disease, it might be difficult for them to recognize you, and you become confused like "Hell no, this is not the Papa San I used to know". Well, that is what Alzheimer's does to you.

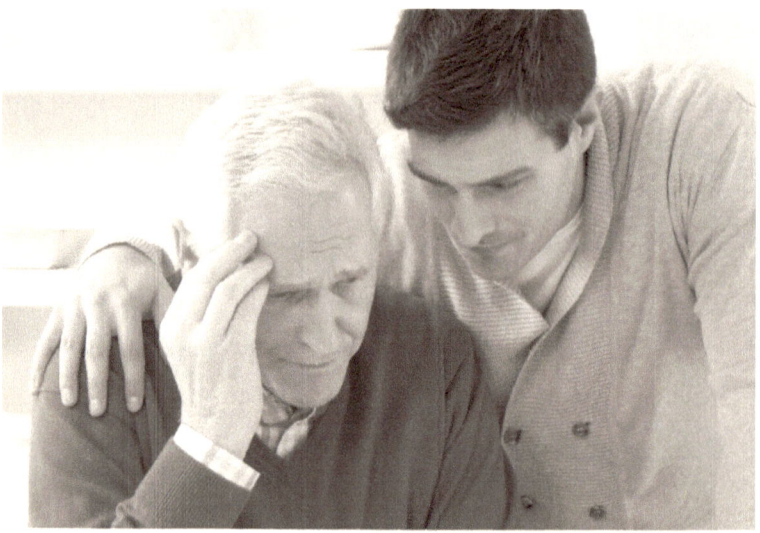

Other effects of Alzheimer's on the seniors include the following:

1. *Their Personality and Behavioral pattern are affected:* This disease turns our seniors to become who they were not in the earlier phases of their lives. A wholly nice and confident person over time changes to become a person with irregular mood changes; obsessive, compulsive, or socially unacceptable behavior; loss of interest, motivation, or initiative; loss of empathy among others. You must understand that this is not who they are; instead, this is what Alzheimer's have turned them to become.

2. *Impairment in speaking, reading, and writing:* They start to have issues with speaking; it affects their speech pattern, they now find it difficult to speak well. Reading books that used to be an easy thing or hobby gradually becomes a difficulty. Also, writing becomes an issue for seniors as a result of Alzheimer's disease.

3. *Impaired visuospatial abilities:* This comes with their inability to identify faces of people and everyday objects, it also comes with failure to make use of simple tools, an example of this is putting on your clothes in the wrong way.

4. *Reasoning Impairment:* This comes with difficulty to think of common words while speaking, including a hesitant speech; the sense of judgment becomes affected, and errors are made with speech, spellings, and writings.

5. Retentive Impairment: Alzheimer's disease come with a drastically reduced ability to take in new information, and difficulty in remembering previous events. What will you say about a person who couldn't recall the sweet memories of his/her wedding day? What about the circumstances surrounding the birth of her first child? Seniors living with Alzheimer's start to misplace personal belongings, forget appointments and events, get lost on a familiar route, and repeating conversations and questions uncontrollably.

6. Getting shunned by loved ones: This here is common with people living around seniors that have Alzheimer's. They try as much as possible to avoid them and even take them away from the society of people. Doing this usually, make things worse for the senior. Neglecting them is not always the best at this stage of their lives.

7. Death: This is the end of it all, sooner or later, deterioration will set, and the resultant effect is always death.

Control of Alzheimer's Disease

Having had all this information, how do you think a disease as vital as Alzheimer's can be controlled? What are things we must do to keep it under check? Do we have a cure for this disease? Well, we are going to take this one after the other.

One thing we need to get straight here is this; there is no cure for Alzheimer's disease, at least not for now, something good could come along the line as to how to get it cured. The death of brain cells is irreversible, I do not doubt any scientific intervention that research could bring forward along the line, but we need to understand that as of now there is no cure for the disease.

However, different therapeutic interventions are usually employed to make it easier for people living with the disease. According to Alzheimer's Association, care for the illness include activities and daycare programs that could make the seniors living with Alzheimer's feel loved, involvement in support group and services which will make them realize that they are not alone, and also effective management of any conditions that surrounds Alzheimer's like the ones we have earlier discussed.

Drug therapies are used to manage the condition and not cure the disease, some option of drugs might reduce the effect and symptoms of the disease, and help our seniors living with Alzheimer's live a better and improved quality of life.

We need to understand that anyone, most notably seniors living with Alzheimer's becomes less and less able to live independently, as they cannot care for themselves as they used to anymore. At this point in their lives, giving them proper care is essential for them to have a quality life, even while they live with the disease.

CHAPTER THREE
DEMENTIA AND THE SENIORS

As we have discussed in the earlier section about Alzheimer's disease and its effects on the seniors, looking into Alzheimer's disease would be incomplete without taking a deep stance into dementia in its relation to the seniors. Seniors in their old age exhibit different forms of diseases and dementia is a prominent one among them. How well do you know of this disease called dementia? Do you have any senior around you diagnosed with dementia? Can you tell more about what they go through with this disease? I would love you to have these questions in mind while I take you through the journey of providing answers to them so you could relate it to what's happening around you. Let's roll.

Understanding Dementia

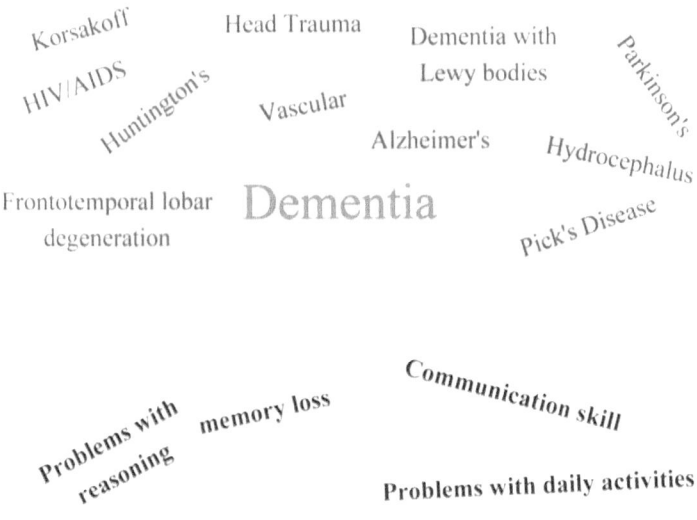

When you hear of the disease called dementia, there should be a couple of things you must keep in view; the source of the disease, the extent of the disease and those most affected by the disease. Moving on from there, we can describe dementia as a large class of brain disease that results to a long-term and usually a gradual decrease in the ability to put your thoughts together, which in turns affects the daily functioning of the affected person. Dementia involves a decline in the mental functioning of a person from the usual way of the proper functioning of the brain. This is what happens when you have a person who is known to be sound in reasoning suddenly or gradually begins to have an uncoordinated reasoning pattern, which will also affect some other parts of the body that will be further discussed under the section of the symptoms involved with dementia.

The common types of dementia include the following:

- *Alzheimer's Disease:* This disease is characterized by what we call plaques, which are found between the dying cells in the brain, and tangles found within the cells of the brain. The presence of the plaques and tangles are to show a form of protein abnormalities in the brain cells structure. The brain tissue of someone living with Alzheimer's disease has fewer nerve cells and connections increasingly, with the total brain size continually shrinking.

- *Mixed Dementia:* This form of dementia shows diagnosis of two or three types occurring together. An example is when a person shows a symptom of Alzheimer's disease and vascular dementia at the same time.

- *Dementia with Lewy Bodies:* It is a neurodegenerative condition that is linked to the abnormalities in the structure of the brain. The brain changes in this situation have involvement of a protein called alpha-synuclein.

- *Parkinson's Disease:* It is a form of dementia that is also marked by the existence of Lewy bodies. In as much as Parkinson's disease is usually considered as a disorder of movement, the symptoms associated with Parkinson can lead to Dementia symptoms.

- *Huntington's Disease:* This form of dementia is characterized by specific types of uncontrolled movements, which also includes dementia.

Other disorders could lead to Dementia symptoms, which includes:

- **Normal Pressure Hydrocephalus:** This occurs when excess cerebrospinal fluid accumulates in the brain.

- **Frontotemporal Dementia:** This type of dementia is also known as Pick's disease.

- **Posterior Cortical Atrophy:** This resembles changes noticed in Alzheimer's disease, but it occurs in a different part of the brain.

- **Down Syndrome:** This is a disease that affects the younger folks, and it increases the likelihood of young-onset Alzheimer's.

Did you notice that all the types of Dementia that I mentioned above involves specifying some scientific terms? Most people are always bored with seeing scientific terms, by identifying this will increase your scope of knowledge towards having a clear understanding of what dementia is all about. I can assure that if you were patient enough to go through those types, you are no longer a lay man.

Moving on from there, we should know that Alzheimer's is the most common type of dementia, which is known to make up of up to 50% – 80% of the cases of dementia. Like Alzheimer's disease, Dementia disease is also a disease that could be exhibited as a resultant effect of aging. This is because it makes seniors highly susceptible to the condition called dementia. It is possible to have the existence of more than one type of dementia in the same person. From a global view, dementia has affected an estimated population of 47.5 million people worldwide. From this population, about 10% of the people develop the disease at some point in their lives, although it becomes more prevalent with age. About 3% of the people have dementia between the ages of 65 – 74 years, 19% have dementia between the ages of 75 -84 years, while close to 50% of those over the age of 85 years have dementia. According to Alzheimer's society, there are around a population of 850,000 people living with Dementia in the United Kingdom, and it is projected that by 2025, the number of people living with dementia in the UK will have increased to around 1 million. An analysis conducted from the most recent census in the United States shows that 4.7 million people were living with Alzheimer's disease (a prominent type of dementia). It should also be noted that there one new case of dementia is diagnosed every 4 seconds; and in as much dementia is not a normal part of aging, the sets of people that it affects most are the older people.

Causes of Dementia

If you would agree with me, to any effect of an action, there are always causes resulting in that action. This is the same way some noted causes could be responsible for dementia, and mind you, dementia can be caused by the death of brain cell, and neurodegenerative disease. We cannot say for now if dementia causes the death of brain cells, or death of brain cell causes dementia. Dementia can be caused by the following:

- *Vascular Dementia:* This is also called multi-infarct Dementia. It happens as a result of the death of brain cells caused by such a condition as a cerebrovascular disease; an example of this is a stroke. It prevents normal blood flow, depriving brain cells of oxygen.

- *Injury:* Injury is a causal agent of post-traumatic dementia that is directly linked to the death of brain cell. Some types of traumatic brain injury – most especially repetitive ones such the ones acquired from sporting activities by sportsmen have been related to some forms of dementia happening to them later in life.

Other causes of dementia include:

- *Prion Diseases:* Example of this is Creutzfekdt-Jakob disease. https://www.cdc.gov/prions/index.html

- *HIV Infection:* There is no certainty to how the virus damages the brain, but it is identified to ensue.

Stages and Associated Symptoms

The stages and associated symptoms of dementia are grouped into four stages, which includes:

- *Mild Cognitive Impairment:* This stage is characterized by general forgetfulness. This stage affects many people as they age, this, however, progresses to dementia for some people.

- *Mild Dementia:* It is observed that people living with dementia at this stage will experience cognitive impairments that occasionally affects their daily life. Symptoms in this stage include confusion, memory loss, getting lost, personality changes, and difficulty in planning and carrying out tasks.

- *Moderate Dementia:* At this stage, daily life for people living with dementia becomes more challenging, and Dementia patients at this phase need more help than ever before. Symptoms at this stage are similar to mild dementia, only that those symptoms become intense. You might need to help the senior in your care get dressed and even comb their hair. Changes in personality may also occur at this stage; they will start getting suspicious and unnecessarily agitated for no reason. Sleep disturbances also happen at this stage.

- *Severe Dementia:* This is the final stage of dementia, and at this stage, symptoms get considerably worsened. There may be an impairment in communication, and at this point, the patient needs full-time care. Bladder control may be lost and sitting and holding one's head up becomes difficult. What happens in the long run for anyone at this stage of dementia is death. It is only a matter of time.

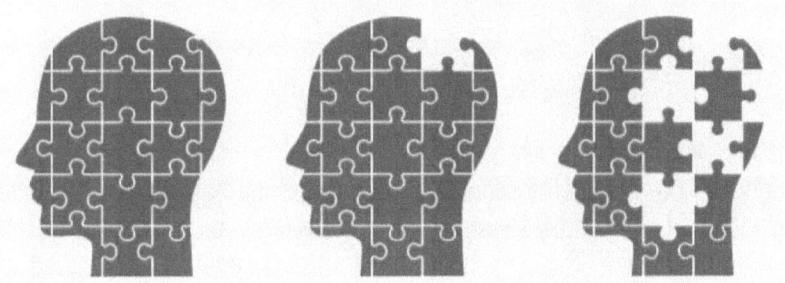

The general symptoms associated with dementia include the following:

- *Difficulty completing accustomed tasks:* People living dementia often find it arduous to do regular duties that they used to, examples involve cooking a meal, making a drink, or cleaning the house.

- *Recent memory loss:* This symptom might be accompanied by the patient asking the same question that had already been answered repeatedly. This is because the retentive memory that used to be there before now is lost.

- **Misplacing things:** People living with dementia at this stage often forget where they place everyday items such as phones, keys, or wallets.

- **Problems with abstract thinking:** They are always not putting their thoughts in place, people these symptoms often have issues when it comes to dealing with money.

- **Communication problems:** This symptom goes in line with the Dementia patients having a speech impairment, forgetting simple words, wrong use of words, and difficulty with language.

- **Loss of initiative:** They don't show interest in getting things done; they are always laid back and not wanting to initiate a course of action that could involve starting something or going somewhere.

- **Personality changes:** This symptom shows people used to know to start exhibiting some attitudes that would make you doubt whether you still recognize them or not. They become irritable, suspicious, fearful, and they lack empathy.

- **Mood swings:** They often switch moods unexpectedly and surprisingly. You notice an unexplained change in their outlook or temper.

Diagnosis

It is like Alzheimer's; there is no one test to determine whether someone has dementia. Medical doctors diagnose dementia based on a careful examination of the medical history, physical examination, laboratory tests, specific changes in thinking, daily function, and behavior associated with each Dementia type. Dementia is examined by medical doctors based on a high level of certainty. However, it is more tasking to determine the particular type of dementia. This is as a result of the fact that the symptoms and brain changes associated with dementia can overlap. For some situations, a doctor may diagnose the disease dementia without mentioning the particular type of dementia that the diagnosis belongs.

It has been shown from studies that dementia cannot be reliably diagnosed without using the standard tests below. After fully completing them, and recording all the answers, then the diagnosis can be made effectively.

The cognitive Dementia tests include some standard intentional questions which are asked below:

- What is your age?
- What is the year?
- What is the time, to the nearest hour?
- What is the name of the hospital where you are present?
- What is your date of birth?
- Can you recognize these people, for example, a family, the doctor, the nurse, or a caregiver?
- Who is the president of your country?
- What is your address?
- Repeat an address of the test that I will give you now (for example, 21, Kensington drive).
- Count in descending order from 20 down to 1.

The results from gathered from these questions are going to be a signifi-cant determinant of giving a correct diagnosis of the presence and the stage of the disease.

Effects of Dementia on the Seniors

The effects of dementia are on the seniors is the same as that of Alzheimer's, wouldn't be wrong to revise it again under this section, would it? Now let's see how bad it could be on the seniors.

1. *Speaking, reading, and writing impairment:* They start to have issues with speaking; it affects their speech pattern; they now find it difficult to speak well. Reading books that used to be an easy thing or hobby gradually becomes a difficulty. Also, writing becomes an issue for seniors as a result of dementia.

2. *Their Personality and Behavioral pattern are affected:* This dis-ease turns our seniors to become who they were not in the earlier phases of their lives. A wholly friendly and confident person over time changes to become a person with irregular mood changes; ob-

sessive, compulsive, or socially unacceptable behavior; loss of interest, motivation, or initiative; loss of empathy among others. You must understand that this is not who they are; instead, this is what dementia have turned them to become.

3. **Reasoning Impairment:** This comes with difficulty to think of common words while speaking, including a hesitant speech; the sense of judgment becomes affected, and errors are made with speech, spellings, and writings.

4. *Impaired visuospatial abilities:* This comes with their inability to identify faces of people and everyday objects, it also comes with failure to make use of simple tools, an example of this is putting on your clothes in the wrong way.

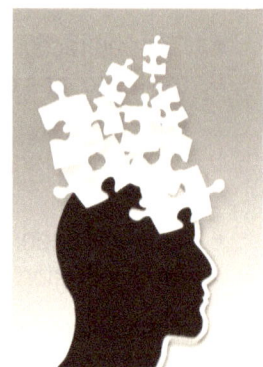

5. **Retentive Impairment:** Dementia disease comes with a drastically reduced ability to take in new information, with difficulty in remembering previous events. What will you say about a person who couldn't recall the sweet memories of his/her wedding day? What about the circumstances surrounding the birth of her first child? Seniors living with dementia start to misplace personal belongings, forget appointments and events, get lost on a familiar route, and repeat conversations and questions uncontrollably.

6. **Getting shunned by loved ones:** This here is common with people living around seniors that have dementia. They try as much as possible to avoid them and even take them away from the society of people. Doing this usually, make things worse for the senior. Neglecting them is not always the best at this stage of their lives.

7. **Death:** This is the end of it all, sooner or later, deterioration will set, and the resultant effect is always death.

The Control of Dementia

It is crucial for us to know that the death of brain cells is irreversible, and as of now, there has been no stated cure for the degenerative disease. Now what we need to know here is how to manage the situation so that it will not make things difficult for our seniors, thereby making life unbearable for them. The disease can be controlled if we are ready and committed to going through the control measures.

We need to watch our seniors closely at this point to make sure they are not indulging in habits that can worsen their condition. Habits like smoking, alcohol should be put under severe check. They need proper care at this point and undivided attention. Medical therapies can also be used to mild the effects of the disease on our seniors, always consult with your physician to ensure correct prescriptions.

Brain training is another mechanism that may help to improve the cognitive functioning, and help deal with a forgetfulness which is likened to the early stages. Devices like mnemonics and other memory aids such as computer recall devices might also be of help.

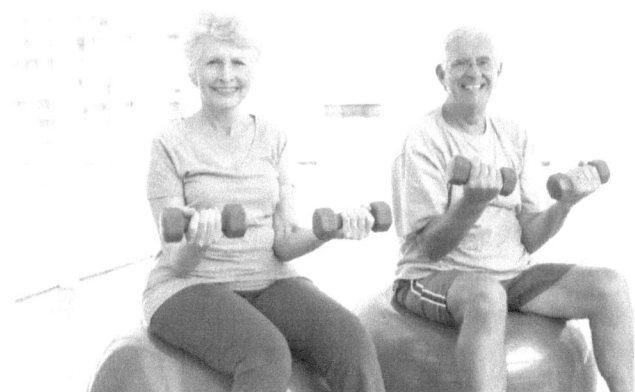

Different therapeutic interventions are always employed to make things easier for our seniors living with dementia. Some of them include getting them enrolled in activities and daycare programs, involvement in support groups where they will meet other patients like themselves. This would go a long way in making them feel loved and make them realize that they are not alone on this journey.

CHAPTER FOUR
ADAPTING TO THE SENIORS

One thing is to understand what the disease is all about concerning the seniors, and another is knowing how to adapt to senior living with Alzheimer's and Dementia. Before you can learn to adapt with your seniors living with these diseases, it is essential for you to have a proper understanding of the disease in line with what your senior exhibits; and if you have been on the journey with us from the earlier sections of this book, then I believe you are on the right path.

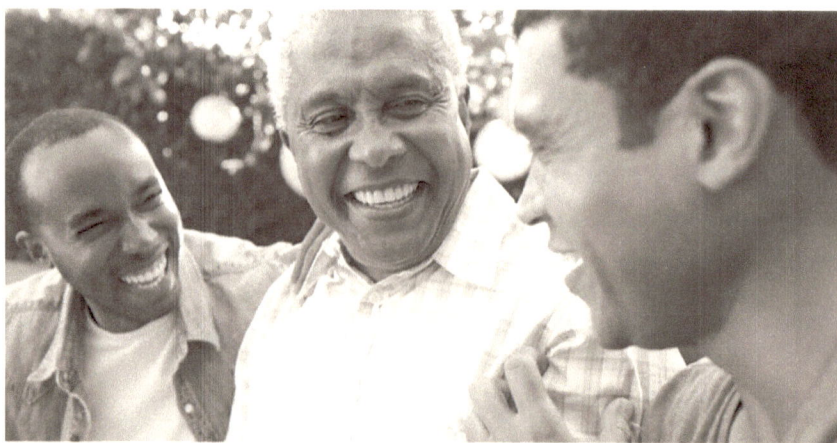

Adapting with seniors living with Alzheimer's and Dementia involves you taking time to study the seniors around you with all concentration and gathering your facts like a researcher would always do before you draw out your conclusions about their situations. This will lead you to help manage their condition effectively, and obviously, you will see the management effects on yourself, on the senior living with you and having the disease, and also on your family who couldn't get a grasp of what is going on. We will further discuss this in the following headings. So, let's move on. Shall we?

Taking Time to Study the Seniors

Beatrice, 52, a single mother with two children, lives with her Mum; Mama Sally, a 75-year-old senior. Mama Sally is loved by everyone in her community due to her active nature when it comes to getting things done. She was a goal getter, always making sure she does everything it takes in her capacity to get tasks done excellently. She never quits. Her favorite adage was "Quitters never win, and winners never quit." Her sense of humor was second to none; this makes her grandchildren and the kids living around her always enjoy every moment they spend with her. Her knowledge of sound judgment makes her preferable compared to a host of other seniors living in the community; whenever you come for advice from Mama Sally, be sure you are going to leave her place with a sound mind to make the right decisions, that's how she is or should I say how good she was? Mama Sally was never alone; she was always in the company of different people; either those she mentors or with the kids coming around to have a good time with her. She was such a lovely soul. It happened that her daughter, Beatrice started noticing some changes in her mother that is quite unusual with the Mama Sally that she use to know. She noticed Mama suddenly started forgetting pieces of stuff, she could keep cellphone on the cabinet in the kitchen, and the next minute she is already looking for it all over the living room arguing that she left it on the table. Beatrice was putting these things to mind, but she didn't consider them as something serious. Things took a drastic turn when Mama Sally went missing on her way to the Grocery store, and she was later found in another neighborhood by the police after Beatrice had filed a report to the police department. All Mama could say when she was found was, she missed her way. Beatrice was surprised at the sudden change. "Common Mama, you've always been going to this grocery store since I was 10," Beatrice said, worried sick that something terrible had happened to her mother. It dawned on Beatrice at this point that she needed to take Mama Sally to the hospital for urgent medical attention. After running some critical examinations by the doctor, she was diagnosed with Middle-stage Alzheimer's. That was terrible news for Beatrice, who is a practicing nurse. Due to her profession, she was able to give proper care to her mother, she made her kids and the people around her in the community to understand Mama Sally's condition and the character that she could be exhibiting under these conditions. The people understood her and were able to give her all the love and support you could ever imagine. Mama Sally was always in the company of people, although at times she withdraws herself from those visiting to be on her own, still the support and attention she got from her loved ones never decreased. Mama Sally was able to live for a couple more years before she finally passed away at the age of 85.

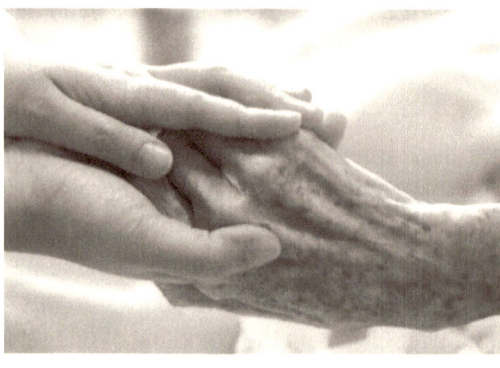

We could notice from this story that the sensitivity of the senior's daughter made her able to see a change in Mama Sally, and was able to understand what to do, and how to handle the situation when she was diagnosed. She knew at that point that it is of utmost importance to study her to understand the ways and manner of handling the peculiarity that comes with her condition. Like it is the work of a psychologist to study human behavior, you need to be sensitive and be calm enough at this point to take time and examine your seniors, you could know whenever they are exhibiting some characters that appear funny. It was easy for Beatrice to adapt because she took her time to study the peculiarity of her mother's disease and the symptoms that she exhibits, and she was able to understand and manage her mother's condition well. So, please take your time to study your seniors so that you can easily adapt to their health conditions, for them to get the love they deserve from you.

Managing the Situation

You need to know that after taking your time to study your seniors and getting your facts about their health condition, the next step for you is to put a well-structured management pattern in place, which will make things easy for you while adapting to the state of your seniors. Managing the situation will involve you informing the people around you of the condition that your senior is facing for them to understand the situation of things around them. And also, for them to know how to interact with the seniors affected with the disease; informing people around you about the health condition of your seniors will make them not take offenses at any character they exhibit as a result of their ailment. It also involves structuring a caregiving schedule that will be effective and less stressful for you. For instance, let's say you have a time demanding job and your senior lives with you, and, I know you wouldn't want to lose the job putting food on the table as a result of taking care of your senior. In this situation, you can employ the services of a trained caregiver that is competent enough to take good care of your senior. However, that is not a good excuse for you not to spend quality time with them. Make sure you plan your time well, so you could have your time giving care apart from the ones your caregiver would provide. When you do this, your face, your voice, and your touch bring familiarity to them even in their period of memory loss when they can hardly remember faces or instances.

Management Effects

To everything that we do, there is always a place of getting resultant effects. When you do what is right, you get the results, same with when you do what is wrong. There is always a consequent effect on each of our actions. What do you think could be the effect of managing the condition of your seniors well? What do you think the impact could be on the seniors, yourself, your family, and the community at large? I know you are smart enough to start providing answers, but, don't think too far, I have alighted some in the subheadings below.

On the seniors

The effective management of the condition of your seniors living with you will make them feel loved and motivated to want to live to see the next and the one after. When you manage their conditions well, you show them the right level of understanding, and they know obviously that in this final phase of their lives, they are not alone. Feeling of loneliness is usually attached to seniors at their final stage of life. They are always yearning for attention and giving them attention, listening to them is a way of managing their situations well and adapting to their condition. When you do this, they are happy and encouraged, and you also give them a reason to fight to stay a while longer.

On yourself

Of a truth managing the situation might not be easy for you at the start, but as time goes on, it becomes part of you, like a routine you must do. You might not believe this, but the thing is, the love you give to them heals your mind and your soul in return. Whether you like it or not, they are a part of you; managing the situation well keeps the bond unbroken, this bond remains even after they have relocated to the world beyond. In addition to this, the scope of your knowledge and resilience increases, and this could help you in other areas of your life. Now you can see that there are quite some significant advantages from which you can benefit when you manage the conditions of your seniors well.

On the family and loved ones

Managing the situation will allow your family and loved ones have a good under-standing and help them accept the condition in good fate; it is hard but doable. When they do not know the situation, they could take a different approach and the relationship within the fam-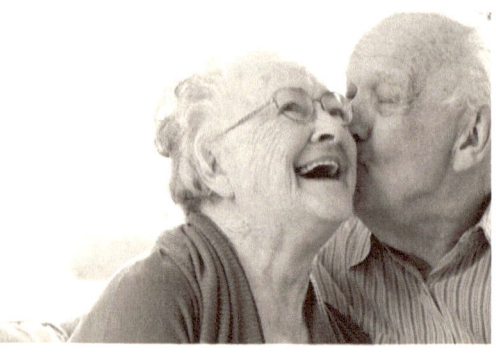ily will become strained. But understanding brings about a genuine love despite the conditions of our seniors and the characteristics they could be exhibiting as a result of their ailment. Managing the situations will encourage family and friends to give support and care in their best way possible, and doing so would strengthen the relationship between you, your seniors, and your family and friends.

CHAPTER FIVE
CARE AND SUPPORT

Let us do a recap of our previous studies here. In the earlier sections of this study, we had an in-depth view into who a senior is, what the traits of a senior are, and what pertains to the phase of being a senior. And we discussed Alzheimer's disease, in line with the seniors, we also discussed Dementia disease; the symptoms of this disease, the diagnosis, the effects, and the control of Dementia. We moved on to discussing the adapting to the health condition of the seniors around us living with Alzheimer's and Dementia; there we talked about taking time to study the seniors living with the disease, managing the situation; and the management effects on the seniors, themselves, and family and loved ones. Now, we are looking at something crucial in the context of this study without which this book will be incomplete, that is the concept of giving care and support to our seniors living with this disease.

Giving proper care and support to the seniors around living with Alzheimer's and Dementia deals with understanding the situation, and knowing that at that point they can little or nothing by themselves, and this will involve our readiness to spend our time, energy, and money to helping through this phase of life. We must be ready to get out of our comfort zone to be able to care and support for those living these diseases. Caring and assisting the seniors might go as far as trying to take them to the restroom to ease themselves and even cleaning them after using the toilet, to help them with taking their bath, and also helping them get dressed, most notably for seniors at the severe phase of the disease. Many people find these tasks challenging to do. We need to understand that at this stage of their lives, they might be a senior, but the condition has turned them to a little child. So, what you need to do is respect them, be patient, take care of them like they are your baby.

The Caring Process for the Seniors

Whatever it is that we do in life has a process attached. There is always a process involved in any action that takes place and caring and supporting for your senior is an inclined action process. Taking care of your seniors living with the disease can be tasking and challenging. If you cannot go through the stress of taking care of your seniors yourself, you can as well employ the services of a caregiver that will be paid for taking care of your seniors. Whether you are the one giving them care directly, hired the services of a caregiver or placed them in a facility, you should know that what are doing is providing care and support to them in every way possible.

However, while employing the services of a caregiver, or facility you should never equate the time the caregiver will spend with your senior as the same with the time you will spend with your senior, However, know that they will cared for an loved. Your senior could be your mother, your father, your grandma, your grandpa, your aunty, your uncle, or even a guardian that adopted you and took care of you till you became grown enough to take care of yourself; this to show that there is a form of bond that exist between you and your loved one who happens to be a senior here. The purpose for placing them into a home, is you might not be able to clean them up after they have messed up their clothes with some quantities of urine, poo or even bio fluids. Always try to be able to visit and comfort your seniors, quality time together, take them on a short walk, push them around on their wheel chair, relate with them on the current level of their intellect caused by the health condition, make them smile in every way possible. That's going to go a long way and trust me although they may forget, you provide the time that was needed.

As a caregiver if you are the one providing care for your loved ones, try and make sure you get a care assessment to get to know what might make life easier while going through the task of providing care to your loved ones. A care assessment helps to recommend ideas to you like someone taking over caring so you can take a break, training in how to lift safely, help with housework and shopping, and also linking you with local support groups so you can have people to talk speak to about in home care.

Alzheimer's

Unknown cause

"Amyloid cascade hypothesis" is most widely discussed and researched hypothesis today

Irreversible

There are no drugs that can cure Alzheimer's, we can only improve symptoms or slow progression

Dementia

Many causes

Diseases, stroke, thyroid issues, vitamin deficiences, reactions to medications, and brain tumors

Potentially reversible

some forms of dementia can be reversed and managed, such as those caused by drugs/alcohol & metabolic disorders

Check out the following caring process for the seniors living with these diseases and exhibiting the following symptoms

Forgetfulness and Gradual Memory loss

In the early stages of Alzheimer's and Dementia, most of your seniors who have this disease can take care of themselves and enjoy life the way they use to before they got diagnosed. But as the symptoms get worse, the people tend to feel anxious, stressed, and scared at not being able to re-member things, follow conversations, or even the ability to concentrate. This is always a difficult period for the seniors as this could bring them to an emotional breakdown and make matters worse for them. Your care and support will go a long way at this time. When their memory starts to fail them at this time, you should always let them accompany you while you help them with everyday tasks such as shopping, laying the table, garden-ing, taking the dog for a walk, and other less stressful chores. Doing this could aid their memory. Also, memory aids used around the will help the seniors remember where things are. You can try putting labels and signs on the fridge, cupboard, drawers, and doors to aid them in remembering what they could have forgotten.

Inordinate Feeding Pattern

Caring for the seniors also involve helping them with their feeding pattern, you need to help them with eating a healthy, balanced diet, as we should note that people with Dementia may not drink enough because they don't even realize that they are thirsty. Not taking enough fluids puts them at risk of urinary tract infections (UTIs), constipation, headaches, among others. They also have common food problems of not recognizing foods, refusing or spitting out food, forgetting what food and drink they like, asking for strange food combinations; this could be as a result of different reasons such as confusion, pain in the mouth caused by sore gums or ill-fitting dentures or sore throats, which create a form of difficulty in chewing and swallowing. You can help by setting aside enough time for meals, providing finger foods if the person struggles with using cutlery, try giving food with stronger flavors and sweeter foods due to their taste buds, offer foods that you they like in smaller portions, and offer fluids in a clear glass or colored cup that they can find it easy to hold.

Using the Toilet

Seniors living with Alzheimer's and Dementia often experience difficulties with using the toilet. These may be as caused by urinary tract infections (UTIs), constipation, which can cause added pressure on the bladder, side reaction from medications, among other causes. They sometimes forget the need for them to go toilet or even not to know the direction to the bathroom, some of them are left with no choice than to pass it out on their body. That could be disgusting. I know, right. As hard as this could be, you help them out by putting signs on the toilet, keeping the toilet door open and keeping a light on at night - having a sensor light wouldn't be a bad idea, studying their body signs and body reactions whenever they need to use the toilet – some of them give uncomfortable and restless looks, or they shake or clamp their thighs, try and keep them active – daily walk helps them with regular bowel movements, you can also make visiting the toilet a routine. The use of waterproof bedding and incontinence pads wouldn't be a bad idea.

Washing and Bathing

People living with Dementia usually become anxious about personal hygiene, and this will bring them to needing a wash. Frequently, have issues with the noisy rush of water from an overhead shower, bath water appear-ing too deep for them, the fear of falling in the bathroom, and being em-barrassed at getting undressed in front of someone else, even if the per-son is your partner. You can help them by asking them how they would prefer to be supported, reassuring them that they won't get hurt, using a bath seat or handheld shower, using the shampoo, soap, or shower gel that the senior prefers, and you should also be prepared to stay with them if they do not want you to leave them alone.

Inordinate Sleeping Pattern

Problems with sleep are one thing that affects seniors living with Alzheimer's and Dementia. They tend to get up repeatedly during the night and may lose their sleep orientation as a result of that. You can help by making sure the senior has a good number of daylight and physical ac-tivities during the day, limit their daytime naps if possible, stop the intake of caffeine and alcohol in the evenings, and also making sure that the bedroom is comfortable – you can either have a night light or blackout blinds. Local services in your area are always willing to support:

- Department of Social Services
- Department of Aging and Disability
- Local Assisted Living homes or facilities (One on One care is al-ways best)
- Local Hospitals and Doctors office can provide additional resources

SUMMARY

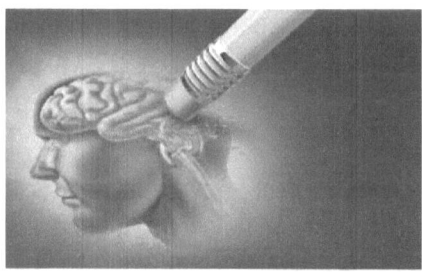

Alzheimer's and Dementia is a challenging disease that affects seniors adversely. You need to understand that when your seniors act irrationally, they are not doing in it intentionally, they are only exhibiting the symptoms that come with the stages of the disease. When this happens, all you can do is understand them and make the people around understand their situation.Giving them support and utmost care at this point is going to go a long way in making them not suffer in the concluding phase of their lives. Take care of your seniors and be sure of a good outcome. Remember that telling them you love them, and you care cannot be equated with showing them how much you care and love them with your constant support and kindness.

The Journey is eternal, thank you for reading!

www.ingramcontent.com/pod-product-compliance
Lightning Source LLC
Chambersburg PA
CBHW020714180526
45163CB00008B/3075